Drive like a woman, shop like a man

Greener is cheaper

Mary Mulvihill

NEW ISLAND

DRIVE LIKE A WOMAN, SHOP LIKE A MAN
First published 2009
by New Island
2 Brookside
Dundrum Road
Dublin 14

www.newisland.ie

Copyright © Mary Mulvihill, 2009

The author has asserted her moral rights.

ISBN 978-1-84840-016-0

British Library Cataloguing Data. A CIP catalogue record for this book
is available from the British Library.

Book design by Sinéad Mc Kenna

Printed in the UK by Cox & Wyman

for my mother, Maureen,

who taught me that the net off the oranges
could be reused as a pot scrub

Thanks

This book has been years in the making – some might say even a lifetime. My thanks to the many people who helped me refine the ideas and arguments over the years, especially: Tom Halpin (Sustainable Energy Ireland) for comments and for correcting some of my misconceptions about energy use; Brendan Keenan (Department of the Environment and formerly of Enfo), for detailed feedback, suggestions and above all encouragement; the many people who took early versions of the book for a test drive; Jonathan Williams, who believed that this was worth doing. Brian, for support (again!) and keeping my bike in working order. Above all, my mother, who is still teaching me how to be green and save money.

Contents

Introduction

You are already halfway there!

It's actually very easy to change how we do things, especially if it means saving time or money – look how quickly we adapted to the plastic-bag levy, and started reusing shopping bags.

So, although changing 101 things may seem daunting, the good news is that the changes are small and easy and, in many cases, we are already halfway there: we turn off the lights when we go to bed, for instance; now we just have to remember to turn them off when we leave the room.

How to use this book

Take 'one a day' and in less than four months you could have saved hundreds of euro andgained some valuable free time, and you may even live longer and healthier as a result. Your wallet, your life and your environment will thank you.

If you do only 10 things, do these

These 101 tips are not the answer to all our problems, but they are a good start and can help you to make big savings. They are not all equal, however, so if you are going to start with just 10 tips, these are the ones to focus on:

- **Get free stuff** (No. 75)
- **Eat less meat** (No. 5)
- **Use off-peak electricity** (No. 81)
- **Get an SUV*** (No. 22)
- **Eat some of your garden** (No. 7)
- **Read newspapers online** (No. 32)
- **Choose what you wear** (No. 63)
- **Eat the seasons** (No. 14)
- **Drink sustainable water** (No. 6)
- **Spread the word** (No. 101)

So, on you go, and keep up the good work.

*SUV: superior urban vehicle!

Preface

Mind your head

Careful! This book could change what you do, and even how you think.

Most of what we do every day is habit: the route we take to work, the way we make coffee, how we wash our hands, leaving the TV on standby . . . Some of those habits waste money, resources and maybe even time. The good news **Rewire your brain** is that once we spot what needs to change we can quickly replace the old habit with a new and improved one.

Whenever we change our behaviour, however, it takes our brain about 21 days to adjust – that's the time needed to build and strengthen a new neural pathway. By then the new behaviour has become a habit, and we do it without having to think. Take any of the tips in this book, put them into practice for three weeks, and you will be surprised at how easy it is to make the change. You'll wonder why you didn't do it sooner.

Allow just three weeks to replace old habits with new and improved ones

What's on the menu?

1. The Goldilocks way to start the day

Forget Oliver Twist and his bowl of gruel. If you haven't rediscovered oats as the best way to start the day, then try food alchemist Heston Blumenthal's favourite: porridge with blueberries.

And why is porridge so good and 'green'? Well, oats are a native crop, grown locally and need little processing, so they are low in food miles, and you are supporting local farmers. There is no added salt or sugar, and oats also help lower cholesterol and blood pressure. They are more filling, so you are less likely to want a snack afterwards. As well as being good for you, oats are much cheaper than other breakfast cereals, and a kilo lasts much longer, so you save bundles, and there's less packaging. What are you waiting for? For a summer breakfast, soak the oats in apple or orange juice and serve with yoghurt and fruit.

Eat more porridge

Gourmet porridge ... served with: Fresh raspberries or raspberry jam, and toasted almonds. A small apple grated into the oats before cooking, and toasted almonds and honey. Raisins and toasted nuts and pumpkin and flax seeds, with honey to taste. Sunday special: a drizzle of whiskey, with honey, cream and hazelnuts.

Basic recipe (one serving): soak a half-cup of oats with a half-cup of water overnight; add a half-cup of milk or water before cooking. Microwave at medium for two minutes, stirring halfway (three minutes, if you forget to soak the oats).

2. Free food

Wild garlic pesto, watercress salad, elderflower cordial, nettle soup, wild blueberries, rowan jelly, periwinkles, blackberry jam, sloe gin . . . Gourmet grub, and yours for the taking.

Our Continental neighbours still forage for and celebrate seasonal wild foods, but we in Ireland have forgotten these delights. Fraughan Sunday is no longer celebrated – the first Sunday in August when wild fraughan blueberries were traditionally picked – and we snobbishly associate wild foods with poverty and famine.

Yet foraging is fun and healthy, free and easy, and the yield is tastier than anything you can buy in a supermarket. Available from April to October, in a country lane near you. Recipes and descriptions in Cyril and Kit Ó Céirín's *Wild and Free*, and Richard Mabey's *Food for Free*.

Release your inner hunter-gatherer

3. What is your 'coke' habit costing?

If you have a soft tooth for soft drinks, it could be costing you anything from €1–€2 a litre, even more if you go for luxury 'traditional' lemonade in a glass bottle. Apart from the cost, all that sugar is hardly good for you, these drinks contain lots of drink 'miles', and are packaged in plastic or glass bottles or in aluminium cans, most of which will probably end up being dumped in a landfill site. (There are also growing health concerns about a chemical, bisphenol A, contained in the lining of drinks cans.)

So why not make your own? It takes just a couple of minutes, contains all the goodness of fresh fruit juice, with no extras, such as the antioxidants needed to keep commercial lemonade 'fresh', costs 50–75% less than commercial versions, and you get to control the amount of sugar. What could be simpler, quicker, cheaper and better for you? And for fizzy lemonade or sparkling ginger beer, you just need some yeast and 24 hours in a warm place for it to brew (lots of easy recipes online).

When life gives you lemons ...
make homemade lemonade

For one litre, you will need: One lemon or two limes, juice and peel (pared with a vegetable peeler); sugar to taste (about 1 ounce). **Method:** Dissolve the sugar in a little hot water in a large jug. Add the fruit juice and peel, and make up to one litre with cold water. Serve with ice cubes and a sprig of mint.

4. The perfect cup of tea

George Orwell had 11 golden rules for making a cup of tea, some of them controversial – he brought the pot to the kettle, and was definitely not a 'milk first' man!* Clearly, making tea is a subtle business, and some cultures have refined it into an art form. In truth, there is only one fundamental rule: if you want a cup of tea, boil one cup of water. No more, no less.

Surveys reveal that we usually boil twice too much water, wasting both *Drink 'green' tea* water and electricity. Given how often we all boil water, that soon adds up. Happily, the solution is easy: measure out the volume of water required, or mark the 1– and 2–cup levels on your kettle, and boil only what you need. There is definitely no need for one of those supposedly green kettles that actually keep water hot on standby!

Fancy a second cup? Then boil two cups of water, make a pot of tea and keep it hot under a cosy. Green or black? Indian or Chinese? Milk first or last? The rest is personal taste.

Measure and boil only the water you need

* 'A Nice Cup of Tea', George Orwell (*Evening Standard*, 12 January 1946)

5. How to save money and live longer

Worried about rising food prices? Happily, there is something simple we can all do to cut food prices which, as well as saving money, produces fewer greenhouse gas emissions, and could even help us to live longer. This simple solution? Eat less meat and dairy products.

The main problem is that more and more people are eating more and more meat – often, three times a day. Rainforest is being cleared to make way for cattle. One-third of the world's crops are now fed to animals – crops that in many *Think vegetarians are wimps? You've never met an angry gorilla!* cases could have been eaten by people. It is all driving up grain prices. Rearing animals is also a very inefficient way of producing protein: one acre of land could feed 20 vegetarians, but only one beef-eating carnivore. Which is why, when it comes to eco-crimes, eating beef is arguably on a par with driving a gas-guzzler and burning biofuel made from food crops.

No wonder the head of the UN's Nobel-prize-winning Intergovernmental Panel on Climate Change has asked people to eat less meat, and to make one day a week meat-free. Others recommend just four portions of meat a week. And what goes for beef goes for dairy: no milk without cows, no dairy products without beef. (Before all the farmers rise up in arms:

we think farmers should produce less meat and milk, but be paid much more for it.)

Switching to a diet with less meat and dairy – and more fruit and veg – is not just good for your wallet and the planet, it's also the key to a long and healthy ***No meat please, I'm driving!*** life and can help keep Alzheimer's disease at bay. And, have you noticed that the vegetarian option on the menu is usually cheaper than the meat or fish?

If you really want meat, eat chicken or pork, because poultry and pigs have a much smaller eco-footprint than beef. Make meat a side dish, not the main one – think 'two veg and a little meat' not 'meat and two veg'. Try organic meat – it is much more expensive, so you'll buy less and eat less, yet savour it all the more.

Eat less meat and dairy

Some stats: Producing just 1 kg of beef generates the same greenhouse gas emissions as driving 250 km in your average European car. Cattle and other ruminants generate 10–15% of global methane emissions, a more powerful greenhouse gas than CO_2. It can take 27 times more energy and 200 times more water to produce 1 kg of beef than 1 kg of plant protein. That 1 kg of beef generates the same greenhouse gas emissions as shipping 25 kg of canned beans from North America.

6. Still, sparkling . . . or sustainable?

How we laughed in the early 1980s, when bottled water went on sale in Ireland. It will never take off, we said. We were wrong . . . in a triumph for marketing, an Irish person now drinks, on average, some 30 litres of bottled water a year. But we were right to laugh – it is a mad, costly, wasteful, unsustainable habit. And just why is water more expensive per litre than petrol?

Q: What's the difference between bottled water and tap water?
A: about €1

Okay, some of our drinking water sources can be unreliable, we'd prefer if our tap water was fluorine-free and San Pellegrino does taste nice. But is that any reason to truck 'couture water' across Europe? Each 500 mls in its own container? Add the energy used in processing and chilling the stuff to the plastic and glass packaging, and the net result is a lot of 'water miles' and a drink that comes with a large dash of 'virtual' diesel.

Maybe you prefer bottled water because most tap water has fluorine and chlorine added? Yet water that spends a long time in a plastic bottle can become contaminated with traces of chemicals from the plastic, such as antimony and plasticiser (added to make the plastic flexible).

Bottled water has the highest mark-up of any item on restaurant menus, so if you don't want to be had, ask for 'sustainable' water. Next time you head out, bring your own bottle of tap water with you. Provide a jug of tap water for meetings. And if you really want to pay for water, then donate to an organisation working to bring clean water to the millions for whom it is still a matter of life or death.

Tap will do nicely, thank you

7. What's that you're eating?

You like your food, right? You like it fresh? You want to know where it's coming from and what was sprayed on it? Are you beginning to worry about eating Kenyan strawberries in December or herbs flown from Israel? You'll be delighted to hear how easy it is to have fresh, local, organically grown fruit and veg for next to nothing right on your doorstep – simply by growing your own.

No, really! If you've never grown fruit or veg before, you'll be surprised at how easy, satisfying, tasty and incredibly cheap it is – a **Dine well, and save money** year's supply of scallions, for instance, for the price of one bunch. Start with herbs, scallions and rocket, which are extremely easy to grow, will not take up much space, don't attract slugs and are much cheaper than any you'll buy in a shop. Don't have a garden? You would be amazed what can be grown on a balcony or even a windowsill, while sprouts and seedlings – watercress, mustard, alfalfa, radish – can be grown on a kitchen counter: all for a small investment of time and effort.

Before you know it, you'll be creating an edible garden packed with fruit trees and bushes, and flower beds crowded with tasty nasturtiums, marigolds, rhubarb and herbs, and swapping some of your broad-bean glut for your neighbour's courgettes. Sustainable, healthy and – arguably – an ethical use of valuable land. What are you waiting for? Start digging!

Eat some of your garden

8. Stop buying lunch

No, not some new diet, or a restriction on your expense account. If you buy lunch at work, even a simple sandwich, it probably costs you €5. That adds up to €25 a week, and more than €1,000 in a working year . . . for food that has been trucked around the place, chilled and packaged, which you could provide at half the price in the time it takes to queue for the sandwich.

BYO lunch to work, and you'll save over €500 – and who couldn't use that! You'll cut down on your food miles and *Save over €500 a year* packaging waste (especially if you use a lunchbox), and you control what you eat. Make sandwiches – anyone for smoked mackerel pâté on brown bread? Take leftovers as salads – roast vegetables and feta cheese with pasta, perhaps? Or reheat last night's chickpea curry with couscous? Or start a lunch club with colleagues – surely they'd like to save €500 as well?

BYO lunch to work

9. Time for dinner?

When someone says 'let's eat', do you: a) get in the car; b) pick up the phone; c) head for the freezer and microwave; or d) take out the chopping board? If you answered a, b or c, then it is time to become a kitchen subversive – and cook your own dinner from scratch.

What better way is there to know what you are eating, and it's quicker than trying to decipher the ingredients on a supermarket meal. It will probably be cheaper, and it needn't take long: fish, spuds and veg can be prepared in under 30 minutes – about as *Get back in the kitchen!* long as it takes to reheat a 'convenience' dinner in the oven – and for half the price of the supermarket equivalent. With fewer ingredients than a ready-made meal, your dinner will also have fewer food miles.

Don't know how to cook? We love the recipes at www.101cookbooks.com. Or use some of the time and money saved in implementing the other tips in this book to treat yourself to a cookery course.

DIY dinner is cheaper, healthier and greener

10. Red, white or green?

Why ship your chardonnay halfway around the world – from South Africa, New Zealand or Chile – when you can sip something equally good that was produced closer to home? The nearer the source, the fewer the booze miles, and the smaller your 'drink problem'.

Some French wineries have even returned to a centuries-old sustainable tradition: shunning trucks and diesel tankers, they are shipping their wine to Ireland across France by barge, and then by clipper sailing ship to Dublin. Apparently, a few days rocking and rolling at sea can improve a wine's palatability. Look for bottles with the Sail Wine logo and an Ecocert.

Buy organic wine, and feel even better: research in Tuscany found that organic wine has half the eco-footprint of conventional wine from the same vineyard. *Sláinte!*

Drink French

11. Irish beer is green . . .

Some of our drinks are very well travelled! By the time
a bottle or can of German beer reaches Ireland, for
instance, it could have clocked up nearly 36,000
kilometres, when you factor in the distances travelled
by all the ingredients and the components that make
up the drink and the
packaging. That's a
lot of 'booze miles'.

And not just on St Patrick's Day!

A beer brewed in Ireland, on the other hand, might
clock up at most 900 kilometres. What's there to think
about? Apart, maybe, from whether or not you should
try home-brewing – which is fun, cheap, has even
fewer beer miles, and is ready to drink in three weeks!

Drink Irish beer

12. Draught Irish is even greener

Beer that comes in bottles or cans is heavily packaged. The sand or aluminium for the packaging has to be quarried, processed and trucked from place to place. Once the packaging has been used, much of it gets chucked in the bin or thrown on the street. Draught beer, on the other hand, gets shipped in reusable kegs – much less wasteful and more efficient all-round. So you know what to order next time you're in the pub.

If you must buy a packaged drink, choose bottles, not cans. Glass has a somewhat smaller eco-footprint than aluminium. There are also growing health and environmental concerns about a chemical used in lining drink cans: bisphenol A (BPA), a 'gender-bending' chemical, or endocrine disrupter (it can, for example, feminise male fish), that is linked with increased incidence of some diseases.

Drink draught beer

13. When there is an 'R' in the month

Rearing shellfish is one form of farming that actually cleans the environment: that's because shellfish, such as oysters and mussels, eat by filtering plankton from the water, and they don't need additional feeding.

Legend has it that a shipwrecked Irishman discovered how to farm mussels in the 17th century: left starving and penniless on the French coast, Patrick Walton slung rope nets in the water to catch birds and fish, but mussel seeds colonised the ropes and Walton later hauled in a fine crop of shellfish. His mussel farming technique is now used around the world.

Rich in omega-3

Mussels and oysters can be grown in Ireland, and are a rich source of trace minerals and omega-3 fatty acids. They need little if any cooking: you can eat oysters raw, and steam mussels in five minutes. Also, they just got greener: the ropes they grow on are now biodegradable.

Eat farmed mussels and oysters

14. Jamie Oliver recommends . . .

Some of our food is very well travelled – like all the chicken meat that now comes from Thailand – but even local foods can clock up the miles moving from producer to processor to distributor to supermarket. Food that travels needs protective packaging, loses nutrients with time and was probably bred to be robust and not for flavour. Imported soft fruits are the worst offenders: often coming by air, it takes far more calories to shift them than they contain. Then there is all the energy used in producing the fertiliser and pesticides, in growing the crop – especially in a heated greenhouse – and harvesting, processing and packaging. Those extras can be significant: tomatoes grown here under heat have a bigger eco-footprint than ones imported from sunny Spain. So, focusing on food miles is only half the picture. But one thing is sure: the average supermarket meal contains a fair dose of diesel.

Don't eat diesel with your dinner

Don't want to eat diesel with your dinner? Follow Jamie Oliver's advice: eat locally grown food in season.*
And support local growers at farmers' markets, where the food is less well travelled and comes with minimal packaging. Also, strawberries are more of a treat when you can only get them in summer.

Eat locally grown food in season

*Rhubarb in April, asparagus in May, strawberries in June, blackberries in September, parsnips in December . . . a calendar of seasonal Irish fruit and veg is in *Dublin's Green Guide* (p191), and at www.dublin.ie (tinyurl.com/68543a).

In the kitchen

15. Get all steamed up

Steam-cooking is all the rage, and rightly so: it's better than frying or boiling, and the food retains more of its vitamins and minerals.

No need to invest in an expensive electric steamer or steam oven, however. Just get a simple stack steamer. You can cook your vegetables and fish in the steam rising from the potatoes, and in heat that would otherwise be lost. It's better for your food, uses less water, and cooking on one ring instead of on two or three will cut the amount of fuel you use by 30–50%.

Stack-steaming saves water, fuel and vitamins

16. Cook like a French yacht owner

Why do yachts people like pressure cookers? Because when fuel supplies are limited, you want something that cooks well in double-quick time. And what works on board ship can work at home to cut energy costs in half.

The pressure cooker was invented in the 1700s in France, a country where they really know how to cook and where pressure cooking remains popular. This venerable technique effectively steam cooks food, preserving the vitamins, minerals and flavours, with **Cook under pressure** the added bonus of cutting cooking times in half. For instance, you can cook potatoes, vegetables and fish (the last wrapped in kitchen paper), all together in a pressure cooker in under 20 minutes. A risotto needs just 10 minutes at pressure, and a stew will cook in 40 minutes rather than the two hours it would take in an oven. The pressure cooker may be old and simple, but it still has a place in the 21st-century kitchen, and is much quicker, cheaper and more flexible than a steamer or steam oven.

Pressured cooked is better cooked

Don't have a pressure cooker?
Try sourcing a free one (See no. 75)

17. Don't be foiled

Which is the odd one out: aluminium foil, cling film or greaseproof paper? Well, aluminium is mined from the ground. The plastic film is made from petrochemicals, which also come from deep underground (it's also a PVC plastic, and can't be recycled). But the paper grows on trees.

The sustainable option for wrapping food? Yes, you've guessed: old-fashioned paper. You can use it to wrap and cover food when steaming or baking, or storing it in the fridge; and after it has been used it can go in the compost bin.

It's a wrap! Aluminium is expensive to
Paper grows on trees produce, and sources will eventually run out, so if you use foil (e.g. take-away dishes, the foil off butter), wash and reuse it as much as you can – for example, to cover a roasting chicken. Cling film contains toxic plasticisers to make it pliable, and if the film is in contact with fatty items such as cheese, traces of these chemicals can migrate into the food. Better to cover the food with a bowl or plate.

Use greaseproof paper, not foil or cling film

18. Cook with less

If a recipe says to use 4 ounces of sugar, do you do as you are told? Or do you rebel?!

Cutting the amount of sugar, salt, fat or oil that you use when cooking is good for your health, your purse and the planet. You'll be surprised how little you can get away with: if it isn't structural (e.g. the sugar in a meringue), or functional (salt is **Less is more** added to yeast bread to kill the yeast cells), then the sugar and salt in a recipe is mostly for taste.

Use half the amount of sugar or fat in a recipe, and leave out most of the salt. The only difference you'll notice is that your ingredients will go twice as far.

Use less, buy less

19. Oven dos and oven don'ts

Forget Darina and Delia, Nigella and Jamie. Here are six useful cookery tips you won't find in their books, but which will save you money.

Don't preheat the oven (unless you are making bread, pastry or a soufflé).

Don't open the door – an oven loses 25°C of heat every time you open the door.

Do turn it off five minutes early – the oven is well insulated and will stay warm.

Do use the fan or convection setting – and reduce cooking time by 25%.

Don't turn it on – use the microwave instead. A microwave is faster, more efficient, and heats only the food (and not also the kitchen and the cook).

Don't turn it on: pan-fry fish, instead of baking or grilling it.

20. Defrost fully overnight

Defrosting something for dinner? You could take it straight from the freezer, pop it in the microwave and defrost it and then cook it, using as much electricity as you possibly can ... or you could run it under the hot tap for an hour.

You could also think ahead, and defrost it in the fridge overnight. This way the food thaws without using electricity and costing you money. It is good from a food-safety point of view (better than leaving the food somewhere warm overnight), and placing something cold in the fridge should reduce the amount of electricity that the fridge consumes. And, when the food is defrosted fully, it will cook faster and use less energy.

Defrosting fully in the fridge is cheaper, safer and greener

21. The great cover-up

Simply putting a lid on a saucepan when you are cooking can significantly cut your energy use. The food will also heat more quickly, and you'll produce less steam and condensation, so you won't need to run the extractor fan at full speed. And, unless you really need to cook on a large hotplate or gas ring – for a wok or griddle, perhaps – switching to a small ring or hotplate can cut your energy use by up to 40%.

Cook with a small ring, a low setting and a lid

Going for a drive

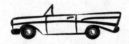

22. Get an SUV

Do you like sitting high above traffic and lording it over other road users? Do you enjoy speeding past commuters sat in their little cars? Want to cut your commute and shorten your working day? Then you need an SUV – a superior urban vehicle.

These elegant speed machines offer unlimited mileage to the gallon, air conditioning as standard, convenient door-to-door transport, quick and easy parking, journey times 25% faster than the 13 kph of city traffic, minimal running costs, plus an aerobic workout while you travel (so you also save the time and money you'd otherwise spend on a gym). And all with half the number of wheels of the average car!

Cut your commute

Back in 2002, the Small Firms Association found it took on average an hour to move a 5-kg parcel 5 km in Dublin, putting us second last in the international rankings, and way behind Singapore's nine minutes.* If only the SFA had used a bicycle instead of a car, Ireland would have topped the list. Cars have their uses, but for short trips – up to 4 or 5 miles, say – you can't beat a bicycle.

Half of all city journeys are less than two miles. Drive, and it could take you 15–20 minutes by the time you've parked the car. Or you could cycle it in 5–10 minutes. If your time is too valuable to waste sitting

* www.sfa.ie (tinyurl.com/3dsjkc)

in traffic then, on your bike, and rediscover the pleasure and freedom of cycling. Don't have a bike? Get one free (see no. 75), or save loads on a new one with the cycling tax allowance. Haven't used a bike in a while? Try Sundays when traffic is lighter to regain your confidence. But remember, a bicycle is not just for children and holidays!

For short trips, you can't beat a bicycle

23. Don't get lost!

Getting lost is a great way to waste time. Driving around lost is a great waste of fuel and money. This is why more and more commercial companies and organisations are investing in satellite navigation (sat-nav) technology to make sure that their fleet drivers know where they are going. The British Metropolitan Police, for example, save about £125,000 a year in fuel costs by not getting lost. Hauliers can save time, and emissions, simply by planning routes *Plan your journey* that avoid time-consuming right-hand turns. Airlines and shipping companies use satellite navigation to plot the cheapest, most fuel-efficient routes.*

You don't have to invest in expensive satellite technology: just ask for directions in advance, consult a map, or use an online route planner, such as viamichelin.com and route.rac.co.uk.

Use a sat-nav or map, save time and fuel

* *New Scientist* enviromental blog (tinyurl.com/3m7lnp)

24. Learn from Ryanair

You might not think that motorists have much to learn from Ryanair. Yet the low-fares airline knows a thing or two about saving money, including the cost of carrying extra fuel. Extra fuel adds to the weight of any vehicle, so it makes fuel-efficiency and environmental sense to carry as little as possible. This is why Ryanair asks pilots to minimise the amount of fuel carried in their planes, and why motorists should take on board Ryanair's recommendation.

Petrol is cheaper by the half-tank

Driving with a full tank of petrol means you get fewer kilometres per litre. If the price of petrol dropped after, say, the first 25 litres, then it might make sense to bulk-buy. But it doesn't. Instead, your fuel efficiency drops. Put another way: bulk-buying costs you money. So, don't fill her up – it is cheaper and cleaner to half-fill the tank instead.

Become a 'low-fares' motorist

25. Double your fuel efficiency

Fuel efficiency is traditionally measured in either miles per gallon or litres per 100 kilometres. When it comes to city traffic, however, we need to factor in how many people are being transported. During rush-hour, most cars carry just the driver – *Join 500,000 French people* probably the most inefficient way of moving one person that our sophisticated high-tech society has yet devised. Happily, motorists can double their fuel efficiency very simply by carrying a passenger.

Interestingly, people drive less aggressively and more safely when they have a passenger. This means fewer crashes, and it helps to keep down insurance and related costs. Car pooling is very popular in France, especially to cut the costs of long-distance routes.

Useful sites:
carpool.ie
dublintraffic.ie/Carpool
gumtree.ie/dublin/rideshare
carshare.com
swiftcommute.ie
covoiturage.fr
liftshare.org (UK site)

So, next time you're driving somewhere, see if a friend can share the ride. And if you have a regular commute, how about car pooling? You share the driving with someone, reduce stress and tiredness, and cut your motoring costs. Many companies provide dedicated parking spaces for shared cars – persuade your employer to do this if they don't already. And if bus lanes ever become car-pool lanes (open to any car carrying at least one passenger), you'll be able to speed ahead of the competition.

Taking the car? Take a passenger too

26. Efficiency drive

Want to save €500 on your annual driving costs? Then take your foot off the pedal! Heavy-footed driving, and cruising at speeds above 100 km/hour can add 30% to your fuel consumption. On an annual average 'mileage' of 16,000 km, that can add up to an extra 400 litres of fuel or more, and over €550. Squeezing more miles from a tank of petrol is a growing cult in the US, where they call it hypermiling.

**Speed kills.
And it uses more petrol**

Anticipation is the key: keep a safe distance from the car ahead, accelerate smoothly, shift into the highest appropriate gear as soon as you can, avoid braking unnecessarily, don't over-rev the engine, and start slowly (give the engine time to warm up). Best of all: leave for appointments five minutes early: you will be less stressed and less likely to rush.

As well as being dirty and expensive, aggressive driving also wears out tyres and brake pads faster, and is more likely to contribute to a serious accident. Smooth driving is cleaner, greener and safer.

Smooth, safe, stress-free – and saving money

27. How to park a car

Question: how long does it take to park a car? Answer: much longer than you think.

Research shows that it really does take much longer to park a car than you think, especially if, like many people, you drive around looking for the perfect parking spot. International studies found that at least 8% of traffic, and often much more, consists of drivers looking for somewhere to park. That adds up to a lot of wasted fuel and unnecessary emissions.

It can take up to 10 minutes at times to find a space and to park. In that time, you could have walked a half mile, saved some petrol money and had some exercise. Factor the 'parking time' into the journey time, and you might find that, for short journeys, it is quicker to leave the car at home and walk.*

Take the first spot you see, then walk to your destination

*Sustrans (UK) report at tinyurl.com/3g8n9a

28. Stop, start, save

When traffic lights in Calcutta turn red, a soothing calm descends on the otherwise cacophonous chaos, because all the drivers turn off their engines. They know that leaving the motor idling while waiting for the lights to change is wasting fuel and money, and adding to the air pollution.

If you have money to burn, then sure – leave the engine running while you are stationary. But if you are going to be sitting there for more than 30 seconds, whether in traffic or waiting for someone to pop back from the shops, it makes sense to switch off: an engine burns more fuel idling for 20 seconds than restarting. Some new cars come fitted with automatic 'stop, start' technology that stops the engine when the car is stationary, and starts it again at a touch on the accelerator. (It makes the new BMW Mini Cooper diesel as efficient as Toyota's much-lauded hybrid Prius, we read in *New Scientist*, and it can be retrofitted to older models.*) Or you could be old-fashioned, and just use the key.

Either way, it is good for the environment, good for your wallet, and good for you. Something to smile about, even in traffic. You'll be surprised at how calming it can be. A Zen moment, even in the rush hour.

Turn off the engine, and relax

*2 February 2008, pp32–36

29. Move up a gear

Driving at 60 km/hour in third gear, rather than fifth, can add a staggering 25% to your fuel consumption. So, shift to a higher gear as soon as you can, and you'll save money and fuel and produce less pollution. Some people recommend keeping an eye on the rev counter – aiming to keep the rpm under about 2,500 (petrol) and 2,000 (diesel) – but I find this simple rule of thumb is easier: 30 kph in 2nd gear, 40 in 3rd, 50 in 4th, and 60 kph in 5th. In other words, most city driving in 3rd–4th gear, and out-of-town in 5th.

Drive in the highest gear possible

30. Don't be a drag, lighten your load

Car designers and manufacturers spend millions creating aerodynamic vehicles. Then we negate all their hard work by adding a roof rack.

The extra 'drag' makes it harder for the car to move through the air, and pushes fuel consumption up significantly, especially at cruising speeds of 80km/hour or more. Carrying an empty roof rack can add 10% (some say as much as 40%) to your fuel consumption, and even the attachment bars on their own add 2%. Likewise, stuff left in the boot is extra weight that adds extra fuel and pollution over a year's motoring.

Clutter could cost you €100 a year

It takes only a few minutes to remove things, and could save you €100 a year.

De-clutter the car

31. Tortoise or hare?

Who'd have thought: slowing traffic down can actually make it move faster. That was the counter-intuitive result from an experiment on England's M42 motorway in 2007: when the rush hour speed limit was cut to 50 mph, journey times improved by over 25%. The main benefits included fewer accidents and a more even and steady traffic flow. Proving that, contrary to expectations, speeding won't necessarily get you to your destination that much earlier. In fact, sometimes slower gets there quicker. Remember the fable? The tortoise beat the hare.

Driving above the speed limit also increases drag and reduces fuel efficiency, so you get fewer miles from your tank and pay more for your journey. It's also illegal, and more likely to cause a serious accident.

Slow and steady wins the race

The life you lead

START

32. What's your news habit costing?

If you buy a daily paper, your news 'habit' could be costing you over €500 a year. That's a lot of money and waste paper (even if you recycle, it costs to make, print and transport the paper and then transport, sort and process the waste). Yet if you have Internet access* you can have all the news for free, and with no waste, simply by reading your paper online. The online editions of *The Irish Times*, *Irish Independent* and *Irish Examiner* are all free, likewise *The Guardian*, and indeed many other titles.

This one tip could save you €500 a year

Reading online does use electricity, but that's still greener than printing, distributing and disposing of newspapers. You'll save time: reading newspapers online is quicker, because you read only the items in which you are really interested. You can always treat yourself to a weekend paper to catch up on all the week's analysis.

Reading news online takes a little time to adjust to, but it soon becomes as natural as email. Try it some Monday, when papers are smaller. Still on dial-up Internet? Save on phone charges by copying the stories you want to read into a document file, and reading them offline later.

Online news: saves time, money and paper

*Most local libraries offer free Internet access, and daily newspapers – perfect for those no longer working 9–5.

33. Want more free time?

We make better decisions if we think ahead. Decide something on impulse now and you're likely to choose, for instance, to eat chocolate or crisps rather than fruit. That's because we all have something of a split personality: thinking about the future engages the rational part of our brain and makes for sensible decision-making; whereas thinking about what to do now engages the brain's impatient – 'reptilian' – dopamine system, the same part that is involved in addiction, and likes chocolate and crisps and the TV-equivalent of fast food.

Engage with your rational self

How to exploit this phenomenon to create more free time? By planning your TV viewing. Next time you buy a weekend paper with the week's TV schedule, let the 'rational you' plan your viewing and mark the programmes you want to watch. Stick to even half of those decisions and you will watch less television and release loads of free time for yourself. Chocolate and crisps are another thing – but planning, with a shopping list, can help there too.

Save time and electricity – plan your TV viewing

34. Share this book

Let's face it: you're only going to read most books once. So why waste money buying a book, when you can borrow it for free from a library or friend? Those '3 for 2' offers from bookshops that would have you buy more books than you need? Well, you know what to do with them. The '8 for 3' offer at your local library (eight books for three weeks, renewable) is much better. You will also be supporting local resources, facilities and jobs, and you can avail of free Internet and daily newspapers while you are there.

Buying second-hand is another useful and money-saving way of sharing and recycling. Books you no longer need can be 'liberated' in a local charity shop or library, or by 'bookcrossing'. That goes for DVDs too.

Of course, you'll want to read this book several times, but once you have implemented all 101 tips, feel free to pass it on. After all, it's good to share.

Join your local library

See:
www.library.ie
www.bookcrossing.com
www.bookswap.ie
www.readitswapit.co.uk

35. Opt out

If you don't want it, then there is no point anyone sending it to you.

Opt out of junk mail and unsolicited leaflets. You will be grateful. So will your post person (their bag will be lighter). And the companies sending the mail (they won't be wasting money on something you're not going to read). And the environment (less junk is less waste).

Opt out of junk mail now

How to ...
Contact the Mailing Preference Service run by the Irish Direct Marketing Association (tel: 01 830-4752), and ask to be removed from Irish marketing databases (you have to contact overseas companies individually yourself).

Tick the 'opt out box' in the Register of Electors – another source of names and addresses for marketing companies. Watch for similar 'opt out boxes' when you fill in forms such as product guarantees.

Contact your telephone service provider to bar unsolicited phone calls and unsolicited mail.

Put a 'No junk mail' sign on your letterbox to cut down on advertising leaflets. And return that *Reader's Digest* special offer 'to sender', asking them to take you off their database.

36. Don't get affluenza

Remember when you were young, and you had a favourite toy, and the more battered it got, the more you loved it? You would never have swapped it for anything, especially not for a new and improved model.

Now, when you get a new gadget or piece of kit – a mobile phone, say, or computer – you love it too, but only until the next 'new and improved' version comes out. Then it's 'out with the old, and in with the new'. It's little more than 'consumer adultery'.

Enough is enough!

The average lifespan of a mobile phone is now about a year. Yet if the old model is still working, why change it? Don't fall for the marketing blurb. Don't listen to those ads. Don't be a neophiliac. Don't add to the growing mountain of electronic waste and unloved, unwanted goods.

Love the model you have

37. Pee for relief

If your toilet dates from pre-1995, then chances are it wastes a lot of good quality drinking water every time you flush it. Modern, slim-line cisterns and dual-flush toilets make do with 4–6 litres, but older models can use anything up to 13 litres. That's a lot of water down the drain every day. In fact, an estimated one-third of Irish drinking water is used for flushing toilets. Water that had to be treated, stored and pumped only to be flushed down the drain.

A quick and simple remedy is to put something in the cistern to displace 1–2 litres and save some water with every flush. You can ***Save as you flush*** buy a fancy folding Hippo bag,* but a simple brick or a litre bottle full of water will suffice. Either way, if you have an older toilet, then just put something in the cistern now.

Put a brick in your loo

*www.hippo-the-watersaver.co.uk

38. Help your bank to save money

Now, this is a bit like hotels asking us to reuse our towels and do our bit for the environment – when really, we think, it is about reducing their laundry costs. But still, there are environmental benefits. Likewise, banks that encourage customers to switch to e-statements: they save all those printing and postage costs, and all the time involved trundling sackloads of envelopes around. In return you now pay for the electricity to download, read and store the electronic statement. But again, there are environmental benefits.

British utility companies have begun charging customers for paper bills. When that practice arrives here, switching to e-billing will save you money. In the meantime, if you do switch to electronic statements, ask your bank to pledge a charitable donation in return.

Move to electronic bank statements and bills

39. Recharge your batteries

Amazing how many battery-powered devices there are in the average household. Remote control units for the TV, DVD, VCR and HiFi. All the cordless and mobile phones. The portable radio. All the smoke alarms. The battery-powered toys. The bicycle lights. The travelling alarm clock. Cordless tools. The emergency torch beside the fuse box. Electric toothbrush? Battery-operated, vibrating mascara? If you are using disposable batteries, that all adds up to a small mountain of toxic waste every year.

Happily, there is an alternative: invest in a universal 'smart' charger, if you don't already have one, and switch to rechargeables. Nickel metal hydrides (NiMH) are the most reliable and least polluting alternative to AA batteries (NiCads are less powerful and contain toxic cadmium). The higher the 'milliamp hours' rating (mAh), the longer the rechargeable battery will last. It's a small outlay at the start, but saves money in the long run and reduces the amount of toxic pollution you produce each year. Turn off all chargers when they are not in use – otherwise, they are wasting electricity – and take dead batteries of all types to a recycling depot.

Switch to rechargeable batteries

Eco-holidays

40. Carbon offsetting?

Worried about your carbon footprint? Guilty about that shopping trip to New York? Thinking of paying a company to plant some trees? Wait!

Carbon offsetting is like the plenary indulgences of old: atoning for our (environmental) sins by paying other people to do a penance for us. But it is difficult to calculate accurately how much CO_2 any one journey is responsible for, and then to ensure that the CO_2 remains permanently and verifiably 'offset'; plus, there is more to pollution and climate change than just CO_2. To be effective, 'offsetting' must be additional; yet most current offset projects make economic sense and would have happened anyway, so there is no real carbon saving. If you are lucky, your payment goes to a development aid project; if not, it probably benefits a private company.[*]

Do your own penance

Happily, there is one effective option, and it may even save you money: DIY offsetting. If you ever gave up chocolate for Lent, then think of this as something similar: atone for your air miles and climate sins by giving up something, or going without. Don't use the car for a couple of weeks, say, give up beef for a month, or don't upgrade the TV. If it hurts a little, so much the better. Best of all, of course, is not to fly in the first place.

Do it yourself

[*]Read Chris Goodall's thought-provoking analysis at carboncommentary.com: tinyurl.com/3owcsh

41. Holiday out of season

There's nothing worse than visiting somewhere at the height of the holiday season. All those crowds, the traffic, the exorbitant prices, the extra pressure on the local environment. The more people who visit somewhere during peak season, the more accommodation and services that have to be provided, and that means more workers, and they need yet more accommodation and services. The original quaint fishing village soon becomes a concrete sprawl.

Taking your holiday out of season will help to spread the tourism load across the year. If enough people do it, it should mean fewer holiday complexes blighting the landscape. You have the place to yourself and can save bundles of money on the cost of the holiday. Surely a win-win situation?

Travel off-peak

42. Turn your home into a holiday home

Do you dream of owning a holiday home? A sustainable, money-saving way to achieve that dream is a house-exchange holiday. And, presto! It's *au revoir* to boring purpose-built holiday apartments with the minimum of comfort and only basic kitchen supplies. And *bonjour* to staying in someone else's comfortable home with all you need. Your own home is occupied, meanwhile.

Fewer holiday homes need to be built, there is less pressure on the environment, and you get your choice of free holiday homes around the world. *Pourquoi pas?*

Sustainable holiday homes for free

Home exchange holidays . . .
Intervac.ie
Homelink.ie
Gumtree.ie
Guardianhomeexchange.com
Homeexchange.com

43. Travelling light

Even without EU security restrictions on liquids in
hand luggage, it makes sense to carry small bottles of
shampoo, shower gel and lotions when travelling.
Except that buying small is expensive and, relatively
speaking, over-packaged.

For an 'eco-nomical' travel wash bag: hold onto
old sample jars and bottles, or the ones given away in
hotels, and decant your own preferred shampoo and
lotion for your trip.

**Make up your own travel-sized bottles for
your wash bag**

Clean, mean and green

44. Get your own back on shampoo manufacturers

Legend has it that, in the 1960s, shampoo manufacturers doubled their sales by adding the word 'Repeat' to the instructions on their labels. Well, now you can fight back. Follow this tip, and you will get better use out of the important (and often expensive) active ingredients, as well as halving the amount of shampoo you use.

The key to getting the best from your shampoo – and this comes from a shampoo manufacturer – is to give the active ingredients time to act. So next time, start your shower by *Half-price shampoo every time* lathering shampoo into your hair, but don't rinse it yet. Leave it to act while you finish your shower, then rinse away the shampoo only at the end. No need to 'repeat'. And your shampoo is now effectively half-price!

Lather, leave, rinse. Do not repeat

45. Do things by halves

What would happen if you halved the amount of detergent you regularly use in the dishwasher and washing machine? Presumably, you think the clothes and dishes wouldn't be properly cleaned – otherwise, you would already be on to this trick. But try it, and prepare to be amazed:
not only will your **_Half a tablet is better than one_** clothes and dishes come
out clean, but the environment will be even cleaner (with only half the amount of detergent polluting the water).

Cut tablets in half with a sharp knife, or use half the recommended amount of powders and liquids, and the only difference you'll notice is that your detergent lasts twice as long.

Cut things in half, and get two for the price of one!

46. Fresh air, not freshener

Commercial air fresheners do not clean the air, they just pump out a chemical cocktail to mask any smells. Put another way, fresheners are a source of air pollution – so if anything, they make things worse. The same goes for many of those scented candles and burners. Some of the compounds in air fresheners can be toxic and some, such as terpenes (found in, for example, pine and lemon scents), can react to produce formaldehyde, which is **Air 'fresheners' are air pollution** a powerful cancer-causing chemical. No wonder that in some studies children living in homes that regularly use air fresheners were sick more often than other children. Plus, although aerosol air fresheners no longer contain CFCs, they still contain hydrocarbon propellants (putting yet more chemicals in the air). And don't get us started on plug-in fresheners – what's that about?

If you want fresh air, open a window. And if you need to get rid of a smell, leave a small bowl of bread soda open in the room. Cheaper, safer and healthier.

No scents is good sense

47. Stick to solids

Go to the bathroom now, and check the ingredients on a bottle of liquid soap or shower gel. Top of the list every time is Aqua, because water is the biggest ingredient. In other words, if you buy liquid soaps and gels you're mostly buying water, and that means lots of hidden 'water miles'. What's more, the liquids usually come in either a heavy glass bottle, or a plastic bottle that was probably made from non-renewable petroleum.

Avoid hidden water miles

Happily, there is a tried and tested alternative: a traditional bar of solid soap, wrapped in simple paper. Save the price of a bottle of liquid soap and spend it on a nice soap dish or drainer to keep the soap dry.

Buy bars of soap, not bottles

48. Who needs dusters?

When you can cut up old T-shirts. No need to
spend money on cloths, just give your old clothes a
second life.

From clothes . . . to cloths

49. Boiling the laundry?

Give us one good reason why the laundry should be boiled at 95°C? Or simmered at 60°C? No, we can't think of one either.* And years of experience tells us that 40°C is fine for everything and, in most cases, so is 30°C.

Heating water to only 30°C or 40°C is a huge saving – Proctor & Gamble reckon that dropping 10°C would save £230 million in electricity costs in the UK every year, which equates to about €20 million in Ireland. Most modern detergents work fine at 30°C, plus the clothes, bedclothes and towels will last longer too. Savings all round.

Do the laundry at 30°C

*Okay: an occasional high-temperature wash with an empty load is recommended to clean the machine, and you need 60°C to kill dust mites.

50. Dry yourself with a stamp

Which would you rather dry yourself with: a dry towel, or a damp one? Okay, silly question. Yet when you emerge wet from a shower and start drying yourself with a towel, the towel quickly gets wet, especially if you have a full head of hair to dry. You might even end up using two towels, and both of them probably become so damp they go straight into the laundry basket afterwards. And washing and drying all those towels adds enormously to household energy bills.

Penny-pinching? No, just eco-nomical!

The eco-nomical solution? Dry yourself all over first with a small face towel – or postage stamp, as they are affectionately known in our household – to take off most of the water, and only then reach for the bath towel. Presto! The luxury of drying yourself with a dry towel, and one that can be used several times before it will need a wash. If you rinse and wring out the face flannel, you can use that several times before it too will need to be washed. Luxury, and dramatic laundry savings all around.

And wash fewer towels

51. Boys, want more free time?

Want to have an extra week every year? Want to add six months to your life, and save money? Want to look manly and mature, yet rebellious and non-conforming? We'd all like more free time, but for people who shave every day there is a simple time- and money-saving solution: love the fuzz, grow a beard.

Give up shaving, and you gain at least 10 minutes a day, or about 50 hours a year, which is an extra one and a half working weeks. Enough for all those projects you've been wanting to get to. And if it's okay for the likes of GQ editor Charlie Porter, 007 actor Daniel Craig and the Tyrone All-Ireland team, then it's good enough for us.

Add six months to your life, and save money

No more close shaves

52. How to wash your teeth?

By turning off the tap! Water is good for wetting and rinsing – but not for cleaning and washing, which is why we use detergents and soap.* It is also a valuable resource, and should not be wasted. It takes money and energy to purify and pump water to your home, and while we generally have enough water in Ireland now, that will not always be the case.

Water is liquid gold

You are already halfway there – after all, you turn off the tap when you are not in the bathroom. Now, you just have to remember to turn it off when you are not using the water. And yes, this is also the way to wash your hands. Got really dirty hands? Put in the plug, and run a little water into the basin (www.taptips.ie).

Turn off the water while you are washing

*Didn't realise that toothpaste contains detergent? The white suds are one clue, and check how many toothpaste ingredients are also found in shampoo!

53. Avoid aerosols

Ppssssss! Anyone who has ever used a communal dressing room will recognise the sound of numerous antiperspirant aerosols filling the air with chemicals, just some of which land where they should on the owner's armpit. Seems a terrible waste: buy one of these things and a lot of your money is going on the complex delivery mechanism and volatile organic propellants, and when you use it half of the contents miss the target.

Happily, there are plenty of options that use fewer superfluous chemicals, last longer, are much cheaper and more economical. They are kinder to the environment also, and will not get up other people's noses. Among them: roll-on and stick applicators, pieces of rock crystal (alum), and – our favourite – a light dusting of bread soda (yes, truly!).

Stick to deodorant

54. Olive oil, vinegar and bread soda

No, not a recipe for some weird vinaigrette dressing! But pretty much all you need to clean your house. The trouble with many commercial cleaning products is that they contain nasty and often corrosive ingredients such as chlorine, perchloroethylene and triclosan. Use these, and you won't be cleaning your house, you'll be polluting it! Switch to edible cleaners, and you'll save money and help detox your house as you clean.

Polish and dust with a drop of olive oil, and you could safely eat your dinner off the table. Bread soda is an excellent scouring **Don't pollute as you 'clean'** powder for cleaning sinks, tiles and basins and even burnt pots (but not to be used on aluminium pans). A splash of vinegar in some warm water is all you need to clean windows. Cheaper and healthier than commercial cleaners, and just as effective.*

Use household cleaners that are safe enough to eat

Extraordinary Uses for Ordinary Things: 2,209 Ways to Save Money and Time, Reader's Digest

55. Greenwash

Yes, biodegradable detergents are usually more expensive than conventional ones. But that does mean you will use them sparingly, so a bottle of biodegradable washing-up liquid will last longer. Because it is non-toxic, you can reuse the washing-up water to wash the vegetables, and then to water the plants. You generate much less pollution and there are no nasty residues on your dishes or clothes. Some health-food stores offer refills, which are both cheaper and save packaging, and there is now a range of brands and products to choose from, including Irish-made Lilly's (www.lillysecoluv.com).

Switch to biodegradable detergents

56. The wonders of sodium bicarbonate (NaHCO$_3$)

Many people shy away from using 'chemicals' in their home, but sodium bicarbonate is multipurpose and has amazing powers.

It is an excellent cleaning agent: use it to remove juice, wine and coffee stains, and in warm water to polish silver. As a scouring powder, a little can be used to clean sinks, tiles, mugs and saucepans (but not aluminium ones). 'Bicarb' is also an effective 'odour eater': leave an open bowl of the powder in a room or fridge to remove smells; or dust it like talc under your armpits as a deodorant.

You can use it to tenderise meat. Treat indigestion with a teaspoonful dissolved in a glass of water. Apply a paste of the stuff to relieve bite stings. Combine it with salt for a mouthwash.* Even extinguish grease fires in a deep fat fryer. And that's just a few of its many uses – there should be a jar of this in every kitchen, bathroom and toilet.

Best of all, you can eat the stuff: you'll find it on the home-baking shelves of supermarkets, where it is better known as bread soda.

Buy bread soda in bulk. Use generously

*Antibacterial, pH-neutralising mouthwash:
Salt, two tablespoons (to kill the bacteria that cause plaque); bread soda, two tablespoons (to neutralise the acid that attacks teeth); mix in a 500ml bottle of water. Use morning and night.

The new shopping

57. Shop like a superchef

Want to save €1,000 a year? According to the Environmental Protection Agency (EPA), each Irish household throws out on average a quarter tonne of food every year – twice what our British neighbours waste. That is about 30% of the food we buy, and worth at least €1,000. Put another way, we buy nearly 50% more than we need.

That is a lot of stuff that was grown, processed, packaged, chilled and trucked around the world, so that we could own it for a while, then chuck it in the bin. Yet, a little planning can save money and reduce the waste-food mountain – you just need to think like a top restaurant chef: plan menus for the week ahead, make a shopping list, then buy only what you need. Your shopping will be quicker and cheaper, and you will buy less and waste less.

Save €1,000 a year

Bought too much ...
Cream: freeze it in an ice-cube tray, then add a cube to a bowl of soup
Bread: freeze it whole, or as crumbs
Vegetables: make soup!
Fresh herbs: make herb butter or pesto and freeze

There is a good scientific reason why planning like this is better than acting on impulse: thinking about the future engages the smart, rational part of our brain; thinking about what to do now engages our impatient, 'reptilian' side. Happily, we can exploit this to make better decisions, reduce our shopping bills, and even watch less TV (see No. 33).

Switching to organic could also help: organic produce is expensive, so you are more likely to buy only what you need, and to use all that you buy.

Shop like a pro – bring a shopping list

58. Think big

A 10-kg sack of spuds, or several small bags? Four small tubs of yoghurt, or a large half-litre one? A miniature box of detergent, or an economy-size one? Two rolls of toilet paper, or 12? Check the prices, and you'll find that buying in bulk is usually cheaper than buying small portions. Plus there is much less packaging, and buying big could mean you won't have to head to the shops so often.

For goods that might go off before you use them all – a sack of potatoes, a 2-kg bag of flour, a packet of seeds* – you could 'buddy up' with a friend or neighbour, and split the contents and the savings.

Buy in bulk, and buddy up

*Who needs 650 parsnip seeds? When you can have 50 parsnip seeds and exchange the other 600 for seeds of scallions, lettuce, parsley . . .

59. Shop naked

Do you pay more for less? Do you buy bagged onions instead of loose ones, for instance? Tea-bags instead of tea leaves? Raisins in little boxes? Pre-washed salad leaves instead of a head of lettuce? A tub of fruit salad instead of some fruit? A dozen pre-packed green chillis from the supermarket when you only need two from the Asian shop? If you answered yes to any of these, then you need to shop naked.

Shopping 'naked' saves you money and reduces packaging and waste: loose fruit and veg are generally cheaper than prepackaged ones, you get to pick the ones you want, and you buy only what you need, so there is less waste. What's more, a tub of fruit salad may be several days old and probably treated with antioxidants to keep it 'fresh'. Where you have to print a price sticker for fruit or veg, you can stick it directly on the item, and when you do need a bag – all those mushrooms, for example – remember to keep and reuse that bag the next time.

Why pay more for less?

Buy food with as little packaging as possible

60. Carton or bottle?

Reusable glass milk bottles are mostly a thing of the past, so the choice today is: carton or plastic bottle. Both can be recycled, but the plastic bottle is made from non-renewable oil, whereas the carton is made mostly from sustainable cardboard. With the added advantage that, in a carton, the milk is protected from sunlight.

Buy milk in cartons

61. Green milk, please

It takes three times more energy to produce a litre of conventional milk than organic milk. This is mostly because of the energy used in producing fertiliser for the pastures. Plus, when artificial fertilisers decay in the soil, they release nitrous oxides – greenhouse gases that can be 300 times more 'warming' than CO_2. Switching to organic milk will add a few cents to your shopping bill – but because it's more expensive you'll buy only what you need, and use every last drop, so it will make sense in the long run.

Buy organic milk

62. Shop like granny

Our grandmothers lived in simpler, more economical and more sustainable times. They shopped locally, ate fruit and veg in season, and thought milk and potatoes were convenience foods. What we need now is to think, shop and act a little bit more like them.

One key piece of equipment – at least for town and city dwellers – is the shopping trolley, or a big basket on wheels. Manufacturers have cottoned on, and there are now trendy new designs and colours. So, you can shop local, carry a sack of potatoes home without breaking your back, and still look cool.

Rediscover the wisdom of your granny

Get a shopping trolley

What to wear?

63. Don't wear pesticides

What's the worst thing you can do to the environment? Some might say flying, or driving a 4x4, or eating beef – but wearing cotton clothes is also seriously damaging.

Conventional cotton farming consumes huge amounts of insecticides and other chemicals, and is unbelievably thirsty. Cotton covers less than 3% of the world's cropland, yet accounts for 24% of all the insecticides used worldwide each year. Who would want to wear so much pesticide? Most cotton fields are irrigated, using between 7,000 and 29,000 litres of water to produce 1 kg of fibre, enough for just one T-shirt and jeans. No wonder the Aral Sea is disappearing.

Green clothes that won't cost the earth
Organic and ethical fashion brands, many available in Ireland or online, include: Edun, Shakti and Unicorn, the Hemp Company, Patagonia, Nudie Jeans, Kuyichi, Fable Clothing, Bishopston Trading, Del Forte, Adili, People Tree and Howies.

Eco-bed linen from an Irish company
www.luxurybamboolinen.com

Happily, there is a growing market for organic cotton – everything from clothes to dishcloths – and alternative fibres. Much less damaging to the environment are crops such as linen (which can be grown in Ireland), hemp and, the new wonder material, bamboo. This fast-growing perennial requires little or no pesticides or fungicides, or ploughing (which consumes fuel and generates greenhouse gases), and can be woven into a nice silky fabric. So, your wardrobe needn't cost the earth. The same goes for bed linen.

Try linen, bamboo, hemp and organic cotton

64. A wind– and solar-powered clothes dryer

Installing a wind turbine or solar-powered system can be expensive, but there is one way to harness wind and solar power for free, and save money at the same time: by drying your clothes on a clothes line.

An electric dryer is one of the heaviest energy users in the home – it *Sunlight is the best disinfectant* can cost up to €1 to dry one load – and the heat takes its toll on fabrics. Air-dried clothes are less likely to need ironing, will last longer, and you don't need fabric softeners or anti-static scented things to get your laundry fresh, so there's an added saving. The wind and solar power are free, and the UV light will help to bleach your whites, kill germs and remove smells. Your clothes and your wallet will thank you.

If you really must . . .
- With gas central heating, it is cheaper and greener to dry clothes beside a radiator than in an electric dryer.
- Gas dryers are cheaper to run than electric ones, and produce fewer emissions.
- Dry light and heavy items separately.
- If you have several loads, do them quickly one after the other, not at intervals, since the dryer will be warmer and more efficient.
- Get a dehumidifier: it is more efficient to dry clothes by sucking the moisture out of them, than heating the air around them in a dryer. And, with a dehumidifier you're ready to tackle any flood!

Nowhere to put a clothes line? Even a clothes-horse in a bright room will do, since clothes emerge barely damp from the fast spins on modern washing machines. And if you dry your clothes indoors in summer that will cool the room – think of it as free air-conditioning!

Air-dried clothes are greener and last longer

65. Pressed for time?

Is ironing the laundry a time-consuming chore? Then stop! Just fold your sheets, towels and clothes neatly once they are aired, as you would if you had ironed them. Then put them at the bottom of the pile in the linen cupboard or clothes drawer. By the time you come to use them, they will **Save time and money** effectively have been pressed.

Heating an iron – actually, heating anything – consumes a lot of electricity, so as well as saving precious time, you are saving money and electricity.

Don't iron, fold

66. Don't get steamed up

Okay, maybe you have to press your silk shirts – but don't use a steam iron. They are much more expensive to run than a conventional iron, since they have to heat the water to steam temperature, and are more expensive to buy. It is cheaper and simpler to use a conventional iron coupled with a spray bottle of water or a clean, damp tea towel or pillowcase.

Who needs a steam iron? Not us

67. Get swishing

Buttons and bows, badges and patches, dyes and fabric paints . . . just what you need to redesign a T-shirt, create a unique, hand-made, designer-personalised garment from last year's shirt, renovate the blouse that acquired a small stain, or **'Green' is the new black!** restore the jumper that has worn a little at the elbows. 'Buy less, and style more', in the words of eco-clothes designer Rebecca Earley. Or, as our mothers and grandmothers used to say: make do and mend.

Fashionista? Recessionista! New clothes, without having to buy them? Let's hear it for the haberdashers.

'Upcycle' your clothes

68. Who wants to be taken to the cleaners?

Do you really want to wear clothes that were soaked in a solvent the International Agency for Research on Cancer (IARC) believes is 'probably carcinogenic'? That's only one of the downsides to dry cleaning: on top of all the chemicals, there is that plastic wrapping, those metal hangers, and

Who'd wear clothes soaked in solvents?

all those car trips to and from the cleaners – it is hard, after all, to carry a suit on a bicycle. Spare a thought, too, for the staff at the dry cleaners who spend their day working with that aforementioned solvent, perchloroethylene, aka 'perc'.

Dry cleaners have their uses (at least, we can think of two: curtains and suits), but given the environmental and financial costs, it is worth keeping dry cleaning to a minimum. If clothes just need to be refreshed after a wear, hang them out to air for an hour or two. Wait till clothes are dirty before heading to the cleaners. Return or reuse the unwanted hangers and plastic wrapping when you are there. And do something else while you are at the shops – don't make it a single-purpose car journey. Best of all, buy clothes that don't have to be dry cleaned in the first place.

Choose clothes 'care-fully'

Gift ideas

69. Luxury hand-made presents

What could be nicer than a unique, hand-made gift? Hand-made goods are lovingly crafted, invested with time, thought and effort, and each one is unique. No wonder hand-made is another word for 'luxury'. The good news is: everyone can make these. They needn't cost the earth, and can be quicker than trying to think of and buy a conventional present.

Don't be stuck for ideas . . . A hand-knitted scarf, home-made chutney or sloe gin; a selection of photos, framed or in an album (perfect for significant birthdays). Or try these delicious chocolate ginger treats, which take just minutes to make.

Chocolate ginger treats
Good chocolate 100g (dark, 70% is especially nice)
Crystallised ginger, about 50g (you'll find it in 'home baking')
Baking tray, lined with paper
Clean jam jar with screw-top lid, and ribbons

Slice the ginger chunks into at least half, or into several small pieces. Melt the chocolate (over water, or one minute at high in the microwave, a few squares at a time, and stir). Using a teaspoon, drop melted chocolate onto the baking sheet, about ½ to 1 tsp of chocolate per drop. Place one slice or four small pieces of ginger on each drop. (Experiment with the proportions – I like twice as much chocolate as ginger.) Refrigerate for 30 minutes. Pack gently into the jam jar, with a little baking paper at the top to prevent movement and breakage. Tie the lid with nice paper and ribbon. Best eaten within a week.

70. Say it with plants

A bouquet can be lovely. And daffodils are glorious in spring. But otherwise, if the flowers can't be grown in Ireland in season, then they were either grown in a glasshouse or, more likely, flown in from abroad. Some of them even travel in water, and most are kept all the while in costly, refrigerated conditions. To ensure perfect blooms, the plants will also have been well dosed with pesticides – so sniff with care, always wash your hands after handling cut flowers, and spare a thought for the workers who are exposed to those chemicals.

Wash your hands after handling cut flowers

Options? There are plenty: grow your own flowers; give a pot-plant, fruit bush or herb plant; or have a native tree planted on the person's behalf.

No bouquets, please

71. For the person who has everything

Surprise presents, 'thank you' presents, birthday presents, 'unbirthday' presents ... we all love getting and giving presents. But what to give the person who has everything? Why, something insubstantial!

Tickets for the theatre or a concert, a year's membership of a favourite organisation, a gift voucher for a massage, a plant from your garden, the offer of an evening's babysitting or to cook them dinner ... The list of possibilities is as long as your imagination. These 'presents of mind' do not need any packaging, and will not add to the world's growing clutter mountain. And many, such as theatre tickets, support local jobs.

Give insubstantial gifts

72. Learn from the Three Wise Men

Ever received a Christmas present that you did not like or need? Well, you are not alone. Surveys suggest that up to one-third of the presents given at Christmas are not appreciated.* With Irish households spending on average nearly €700 on Christmas gifts, according to the 2008 Deloitte Christmas survey, that adds up to over €250 million in wasted money and, well, gift-wrapped landfill. Not to mention all the time wasted in crowded shops trying to decide what to buy.

Happily, it is easy to avoid: if you don't know what someone needs or wants and are too shy to ask, then follow the example of the three wise men, and give them money or a voucher (Melchior had to make do with gold). They will make sure to buy the present they want.

Give them what they want

*The Deadweight Loss of Christmas, *American Economic Review*, 1993

73. Christmas selection box?

Selection boxes have become a traditional stocking filler. Yet they can be an expensive way of buying sweets and chocolate, and they come with lots of unnecessary packaging. Cheaper and more 'ecological' to put together your own selection box. And that way, there will be no unwanted bars.

Make your own selection

Reincarnation

74. Cut your waste charges in half

Simple: become a rotter! Stop throwing waste food in the bin, start composting instead, and the amount of waste you generate will drop dramatically.

If you have never made compost, fear not. It is incredibly easy – just let nature take over – and very satisfying to turn waste food magically into crumbly 'black gold' compost. You don't even need a garden: there are small compost kits for city balconies too, and if you don't need the compost, one of your neighbours will gladly oblige.

Teabags, coffee grounds, raw fruit and vegetable peelings, newspapers, raw egg shells (crushed) . . . all can be composted. No meat, fish or cooked food – for those you need a 'digester' cone. Keep a small bin in the kitchen to collect the peelings; line the bin with newspaper to absorb moisture, and it won't smell. Then watch as this simple alchemy turns a waste into a useful resource, and saves you money on bin charges.

Start rotting now

75. Free stuff!

Imagine a place where the things you need are free. A DVD player, child's cot, exercise treadmill, kitchen table, computer keyboard . . . All you have to do is collect them. Imagine another place where you could get rid of things you no longer need – a DVD player, child's cot, treadmill . . . And all you have to do is let people come and collect them.

Well, thanks to the wonders of email, there are now several online communities where you can find a good home for stuff you don't need, and locate a free source of something you do need. Since we joined Freecycle, we've managed to 'freecycle' an unwanted heater, computer equipment, furniture and even leftover plasterboard. In turn we've acquired a DVD player among other things.

'Freecycling' reduces the amount of stuff going to landfill, gives a new lease of life to objects, and reduces the number of new products being made and bought. There's the joy of giving something to someone who really wants it, and the pleasure of meeting like-minded souls. Try it – there's sure to be a community near you. So, if you don't have it, don't buy it, and if you don't want it, don't dump it . . . until you've tried freecycling it.

Get freecycling

Everything is free on...
www.freecycle.org
www.jumbletown.ie
www.dublinwaste.ie

76. Reasons to recycle aluminium

Aluminium is a wonderful material. Lightweight and flexible, it can be used in endless applications, from aeroplanes and high-speed ferries, to cars and bicycles, kitchen foil and take-away containers, and the ubiquitous drinks can. It is, however, very expensive to manufacture: producing one tonne from bauxite ore uses 15 MW of electricity. Fortunately, aluminium is easy to recycle, it can be recycled endlessly, and recycling uses only 5% of the electricity used to produce fresh aluminium from ore. Hence, recycling one aluminium can saves enough electricity to power a TV for three hours.

Aluminium is the only packaging material that not only covers the cost of collection and re-processing for itself, but also subsidises the recycling costs of other materials such as plastic and glass.* Yet only about half the aluminium used in Ireland is recycled – the rest of this valuable material is still thrown away. Shame on us.

Recycle more aluminium

77. Paint the town green

Is there a half-tin of paint lurking under your stairs? If you've ever decorated, then the chances are you still have several half-empty tins of unwanted paint. In addition to taking up space, they are a fire risk, and a form of hazardous waste – you can't just throw paint out, you have to take it to a special depot for disposal. Yet, now it can be put to good use.

The Community RePaint project* takes all sorts of paints, varnishes, wood stains and finishes provided they are in the original container and can still be used. They will *Don't throw it away –* sort and then distribute these to *there is no 'away'* community and voluntary groups in need of a lick of paint. Even that half-tin of deep green gloss can be added to a multi-coloured mural. A win-win situation for everyone.

Donate unused paint

*www.rediscoverycentre.ie: currently available in Dublin only, but watch this space

78. Convert to reincarnation

A brand new car loses most of its value in that first minute when the owner takes possession of the keys. In that instant, it goes from being brand new to being second-hand. By the same token, everything we own is at least second-hand or, as some sales-people prefer to say, pre-owned and pre-loved. Now, some folk turn up their noses at second-hand goods, but strangely, the more 'second-hand' something is the more attractive (and valuable) it becomes. Think antiques, collectables and 'vintage'.

Everything you own is second-hand

Buying second-hand – whether it's cars, clothes or furniture, and whether from eBay or from an antique or charity shop – helps to give something a new lease of life. 'Collectables' also make excellent presents: unusual gifts which, because they were already in existence, did not have to be made anew. Don't call it recycling, but rather 'reincarnation'.

New to second-hand shopping? Well it doesn't hurt to start by browsing. Perhaps you have something you could donate or sell?

Buy more 'antiques'

79. The end of the indium is nigh

Forget peak oil, that's only the tip of the (fast-melting) iceberg. World reserves of indium – used in making LCDs and flat screen TVs – could run out by 2017. Platinum (a vital constituent of catalytic converters and fuel cells) could be exhausted by 2020, and some researchers are already trying to 'harvest' the metal from road dust. Hafnium (used in computer chips) could be gone by 2017, and terbium (used in fluorescent light bulbs) could be all gone by as early as 2012.*

These are rough estimates, and we may discover new sources for some of the rare elements that buy us a few more years. Landfill mining *Reduce, reuse and recycle – or run out* could be the next big thing! But eventually, supplies will run out. And our only salvation will lie in finding alternatives, and recycling the rest.

Recycle – while we still have stuff to recycle

* 'Earth Audit', by David Coen, *New Scientist*, issue 2605, 2007

80. It's good to share

There is something very nice about sharing, and lending to a friend or neighbour helps build relations and even communities. It also cuts down on waste and consumption, especially for appliances that are used only occasionally: no need for everyone in the village to have a power-washer, if you are willing to lend the one that is collecting dust in your garage. And in return, you can borrow a hedge trimmer from the neighbour down the road, and a wallpaper stripper from the folks across the way.

Sharing can even work with magazines – when you've finished with your current-affairs weekly and the literary monthly, you can pass them on to a friend, local school or even GP surgery. Much better to give them a second life than to throw them in the recycling bin. Your mother was right – it is good to share!

Share, and share alike

The power drill

81. Avoid the power 'rush hour'

We can't all install a wind turbine in the garden, yet simply changing when we use electricity can make our power consumption greener. Electricity production is dirtiest and most expensive when demand is highest: 5–7 pm on winter evenings when heating systems, TVs, kettles, ovens and lights come on in every home and every power station has to be brought on stream, including older and more polluting ones.* Conversely, production is cleanest, cheapest and greenest when demand is lowest, especially later at night.

Get a night-life – spread the workload

Spreading electricity consumption across the day could save us all money by reducing the amount of fossil fuels we burn and the number of generating stations we need. Power-hungry tasks such as using the dishwasher could be left until late at night (but not unattended overnight, on account of the fire risk) and we could try to use as little electricity as possible during the busy and 'dirty' 5–7 pm period.

Commercial customers already pay more for 'peak' power, so they can actually save money by switching off things. Domestic customers who can avail of cheaper night-rate electricity can also save – the rest of us will have to wait until 'smart meters' are introduced.

Off-peak electricity is cleaner, greener and potentially cheaper
*Watch real-time electricity demand rise and fall at www.eirgrid.com

82. Save by degrees

Walk over to your central-heating control panel now, and turn down the thermostat. Every 1°C drop could cut your energy bills by 10%. For central heating, 20°C is a comfortable yet economic setting.

If there is a temperature control for the hot-water, then do the same there. There is little point in spending money to heat water to 70°C, only to add cold water so you can use it. It is simpler and cheaper to set the thermostat to *Drop 1°C, save 10% on your energy bill* 50°C. Find the lowest temperature that's comfortable for you, and the cheapest, by experiment: lowering the thermostat a degree or two at a time. In summer, it should be possible to turn it down by several degrees more. You'll be saving money and fuel, and cutting your emissions. What are you waiting for? Do it now!

Turn down the thermostat on the heating and hot water

83. Don't see red

Colin Pykett, a retired UK Ministry of Defence physicist, didn't believe environmentalists who said that appliances left on standby were still using 20% of the power they used when switched on. So he took state-of-the-art monitoring equipment, and proved they were wrong: his cordless phone, CD player and all the other appliances on standby actually used 24% of their full electricity consumption.* And some appliances drew current, even when the red front-panel LED indicated that they had been switched off.

Watts on? If it feels warm, it is using current

Happily, there is a simple piece of kit that takes care of the standby problem, and costs nothing: it's called a socket. Switch things off at the socket, or unplug them, when they are not in use and you will save 20–24% of the power they normally consume, and cut your total electricity bill by 5–10%. We're talking the TV and DVD player, hi-fi, PC, printer, scanner and modem, phone charger, oven and microwave and, when you go away for a few days, the cordless phone. A good test is to feel something: if it is warm, then it is drawing current, and if it is not in use, then it is wasting money and electricity.

Live life unplugged – cut your electricity bill by 5–10%

*Physics World, July 2007

84. Lights on, and nobody home?

Consider the humble light bulb. This invention has lit our homes for a century, shedding light, revealing dust(!), and allowing us to continue reading and working well into the night. No wonder it is the iconic symbol for a bright idea.

Once, there was one bulb in each room. Now there are lots, all on at the same time, many are not necessary, and some are power-hungry halogen lights. No wonder lighting accounts for 19% of world electricity production, and much of that is wasted: empty offices lit up all night, lights on in empty rooms across the country.

If every Irish household switched off two 100-watt light bulbs in the evening – a room no one is using just now, the upstairs landing – it would save 200 MW, equivalent to a small power station. Then again, what is a 100-watt bulb doing on the landing? Surely you switched to a low-energy CFL for the landing long ago?*

Leaving a room for a while? Turn out the lights!

*CFLs are ideal for hallways and living rooms, but less suited to lights that are on intermittently (e.g. in a toilet). Rather than convert fully to CFLs, we await the next generation of LEDs (light emitting diodes), already available for reading lamps and bicycle lights.

85. The full load

Wait till you have a full load before switching on the washing machine or dishwasher. Half-loads are a waste of space, electricity, detergent and money. Ditto the pre-wash soak – try doing without it, and see for yourself. If some dishes are likely to smell (that fishy plate, for instance), rinse them lightly and they should keep until the machine is full. That said, if your machine has a half-load option, then this should be acceptable, since it uses half the water, and the main cost lies in heating the water.

Wash only when full

86. Have you money to burn?

If you have the heating on after dark, but the curtains are open, the blinds are up and some of the rooms are open, then you must have money to burn. Because some of that heat – and your hard-earned cash – is going straight out the window to warm the great outdoors, and some is leaving the room by the open door, probably to warm spaces that don't need to be heated, and generating uncomfortable draughts as it leaves. Meanwhile, the boiler is working overtime just to keep up – **_Draughts can make a_** a bit like filling the car's petrol tank **_warm room feel cold_** while the engine is running.

Save some of your money and some of your heat simply by closing all the curtains and doors once the sun has gone down, and reversing the process by day to let in any warmth from the sun – the cheapest form of heating available! In summer, do the opposite: keep your home cool by closing the curtains to block out the sun – and you will need no air-conditioning.

Close the curtains, shut that door

87. Melt some ice

Ice growing inside your freezer does not mean that it is colder in there. In fact, a build-up of more than 6mm of frost means that the motor has to work harder, and that uses more electricity and makes the freezer less efficient and more expensive to run.

You will have to defrost it sooner or later, and best to do it every six months, before the ice gets so thick that it causes a flood when you do defrost it.*

Defrost the freezer regularly

*Bowls of hot water in the freezer will speed up the process; meanwhile, store the frozen foods in the fridge or the oven (both are insulated boxes) until the freezer is ready.

88. Dress for the weather

Feeling cold? Don't put on the heating . . . until you've put on a vest or a T-shirt and a warm jumper and socks. We live in the northern hemisphere, after all. It's supposed to be cold in winter. And the central heating system is not there to allow you to wander round the house in summer clothes and bare feet.

Dress for the seasons, and you should be able to turn off the heating in April, and keep it off until well into October – saving money all the while.

Put on extra layers before putting on the heating

89. Don't warm an empty room

If a room is not in use, then turn off the radiator and close the door. And that goes for the bedrooms: no need to warm them all day – just turn on the radiator there for an hour in the evening. You will sleep better in a room that isn't overheated and stuffy.

Keep empty rooms cool and closed

90. Exploit your home's insulation

Your home is well insulated – isn't it? So it will stay comfortably warm for up to an hour after the heating switches off. Which means you can safely turn off the heating an hour before – and not 'as' – you go to bed, and an hour before you go out.

Switch off the heating an hour early

Nine-to-five

91. Try a back-of-the-envelope calculation

When office and personal computers were arriving in the 1980s, we were promised the paperless office. Yet we now use three times more paper per person than 25 years ago – 60 kg a year – and half of it is wasted. Computers make it all too easy to print files and emails, and half the time we print the wrong document, or the same document several times by mistake. Much of what we print gets thrown out the same day. There is a lot about the 1980s that we wouldn't want to return to, but at least back then we weren't wasting so much paper.

Give every piece of paper a second lease of life

Set your print options to display a preview first, and you are less likely to print the wrong document. If you read and store an email, you may not need to print it at all. And if you do print a file, use both sides of the paper. Give every piece of paper a second life: use the back for rough work, and cut waste pages into smaller pieces for use as telephone message pads and shopping lists.

Print less, use less, pay less

92. New computer?

A computer is a wonderfully sophisticated device. It contains intricate components, and calls for high-tech manufacturing. However, making a computer also uses hazardous chemicals (such as brominated flame retardants), and many of the components contain toxic metals (such as cadmium and lead), some of which are in short supply. So throwing out an old computer and buying a new one can be a dirty business, and with hundreds of new computers bought in Ireland every day, that pollution soon adds up.

Thinking of upgrading your computer? See can you make the old one last a little longer first (e.g. clean the hard drive, delete unwanted files and software). Buy as much memory and RAM as you can afford, so the new machine will last as long as possible. Read the Greenpeace Guide to Green Electronics, to see which manufacturers are doing their bit for the environment.* Best of all, check out the Irish eco-computer (www.iameco.com) which can be updated, upgraded, reused and recycled and comes in a nice wooden case.

Green wooden Irish computer

*www.greenpeace.org at tinyurl.com/cc4j9

93. Screen saver? Energy waster!

The average computer consumes about 130 watts –
twice that, if it's running a power-hungry computer
game. Screen-saver mode cuts the power consumption
only by 8–10%. Even in standby or 'sleep' mode, a
computer will still be using nearly 25% of its full
power consumption. (Macs are more efficient than
PCs running Windows, but the same percentages
usually apply.) Individually it's not a lot, but think of all
the computers left running all day, every day.

If you don't want to waste energy and money, turn
the screen off and set your computer to 'go to sleep'
after, say, five minutes. And if you're not going to use
it for half an hour or more – coffee break, lunchtime,
when you go home in the evening . . . at the weekend?
– then turn it off altogether.

**Exercise the off button on your computer
and monitor**

94. Be a mug at work

Spurn the disposable plastic cup from the water cooler. Say 'No!' to the paper coffee cup in the canteen. Say an even bigger 'No!' to the cardboard sleeve for the coffee cup.

Keep your own reusable mug and glass on your desk, and save every time you take a drink.

Got my own mug, thank you!

95. Breathe easy at work

The air in a modern home or office can be pretty polluted, with a cocktail of chemicals such as ozone, formaldehyde, carbon black particulates, ammonia, volatile organic compounds (VOCs), toluene . . . These come from synthetic furnishings and paints, cleaning products, and the inks, toners and even the papers used in printers and photocopiers.

Want to breathe easy? Let in plenty of fresh air. Print as little as possible. Turn off the printer and photocopier when they are not in use. **Printing pollutes!** And keep some pot plants on the desk – a NASA study found that plants can scrub 99% of the toxins from indoor air pollution, especially bamboo, which can handle a range of chemicals. (Spider and rubber plants will remove formaldehyde, azaleas will scrub the chemicals emitted by synthetic carpets, while chrysanthemums can deal with the chemicals from fresh paint and plastic.)

Pot plants make an office greener and cleaner

96. Save as you print

You got a nice colour printer with your new computer, right? But does everything have to be printed in 'letter' quality? Do you really need to print your airline confirmation in full colour? And every email and web address in blue ink?

Strangely, the default settings on printers are the ones that use the most ink. You could call it 'a licence to print money' for the printer companies. Two simple changes will make your inks go much further and, since inks are the most expensive thing about printing, this will save **It's not grey, it's green!** you lots of money. First, set your printer to black-only (sometimes called 'greyscale'), to save on the expensive colour cartridges. Second, select the 'draft' setting (300 dpi for a laser printer), and the toner saver option if there is one, and your black ink – and your money – will go twice as far.

Save inks, save money

97. When brown is a shade of green

White envelopes may look brighter than brown ones, but that's only because they are made from virgin woodpulp, and probably chemically bleached too. Brown or 'manila' envelopes, on the other hand, are not bleached and often contain some recycled paper. They are also cheaper, so switching will save you money as well.

Use brown envelopes, not white

Try:
Envelopes made out of waste paper from direktrecycling.net

98. Who needs paperclips?

Take a tip from millionaire entrepreneur and *Dragon's Den* regular, Duncan Bannatyne, and stop buying paper clips. Bannatyne realised that so many paperclips arrive in the post or lurk on people's desks that his company did not need to buy new ones. By collecting and reusing old ones, they saved £5,000 a year, and some valuable steel. And if that tip is good enough for a Dragon, it's good enough for us.

Save and reuse paperclips

99. Storage costs money, even in cyberspace

Storing files and emails online is wonderfully convenient. We are particularly fond of gmail: instant access to all our emails – any time, anywhere – and gmail even provides a very generous 7.2 GB (and counting) of online storage space in each of our gmail accounts. So it is very tempting just to let all those emails mount up.

Store only the files you need

Until you remember that all those files have to be stored on a computer somewhere and, what's more, one that is running all the time. So, if you store files online, you are using power even when your own computer is switched off. Which explains why 3% of electricity consumption in the USA now goes to powering the Internet.

Spring clean online accounts, and save energy

100. The write stuff

Writing is one of civilisation's greatest inventions, and the pen is one of our most important tools. Time was when a pen was an expensive item; now they are given away free. No wonder the world is fast filling up with disposable plastic ballpoint pens, each one of which will take thousands of years to decompose in a landfill site.

This is one good reason for switching to the traditional, refillable, 'so much more stylish' reuseable fountain pen. With a pen and bottle of ink you can write for miles. Then say 'No!' to free pens and other freebies. Nothing is ever 'free', and the chances are you have a drawerful of pens somewhere anyway.

Use ink to the very last drop

Pick up a fountain pen

Spread the word

101. Spread the word

If you discovered a great new restaurant or read a good book, you would tell your friends about it – right? Likewise, if there were great savings to be made in a sale?

And there are great savings to be made here – saving money, time and resources. So, if you like any of these tips – even just one – make sure to tell a friend about it. That way, they can enjoy the savings too, and you double the impact.

Tell a friend about the savings you are making

Sources and resources

A selection of the books and websites, campaigns, communities and companies, organisations and services now available for those looking to do less and use less.

Books

Carbon Counter: calculate your carbon footprint, Mark Lynas, HarperCollins, 2007

Carbon Detox: your step-by-step guide to getting real about climate change, George Marshall, Gaia Thinking, 2007

Dublin's Green Guide: an earth-friendly sourcebook, Dublin City Council, also available online at www.dublin.ie (tinyurl.com/68543a)

Extraordinary Uses for Ordinary Things: 2,209 Ways to Save Money and Time, Reader's Digest, 2007

Go Make a Difference: over 500 daily ways to save the planet, Think Books, 2006

How to Live a Low-Carbon Life, Chris Goodall, Earthscan Publications, 2007

In Defence of Food: An eater's manifesto, Michael Pollan, Penguin, 2008

Saving the Planet without Costing the Earth: 500 simple steps to a greener lifestyle, Donnachadh McCarthy, Fusion Press, 2004

Stop Wasting your Money, Conor Pope, Liberties Press, 2008

Websites

Anti-Apathy (www.antiapathy.org) Worn Again shoes – 'some things are just too good to go to waste' –just one of the initiatives from London-based AA, which supports creative approaches to social and environmental issues.

Carbon Commentary
(www.carboncommentary.com) insight and analysis from 'low-carbon' author Chris Goodall.

CELT, Centre for Environmental Living and Training (www.celtnet.org): courses in skills and crafts, from coppicing to dry-stone walling. Based in County Clare.

Codema (codema.ie) energy and sustainability services, for local authorities and the private sector.

Comhar, the Sustainable Development Council (www.comharsdc.ie) national forum for sustainable development, offers grant aid for projects. Its 25 members are nominated from the state, economic sectors, academia and NGOs.

Cultivate (www.cultivate.ie) eco-shop, resource centre, and workers' co-operative running courses on everything from green building to perma-culture, in Dublin city. Also hosts the annual Sustainable Living Festival. Open to membership.

Cyclists.ie On your bike! Coalition of seven cycling groups campaigning to improve things for Irish cyclists.

Dublin Transportation Office (www.dto.ie) Need a walking or cycling route in Dublin? Try the DTO's route planner.

ÉASCA (www.easca.ie) the Environmental and Sustainable Construction Association promoting sustainable construction in Ireland.

Eat the Seasons (www.eattheseasons.co.uk) What's good to eat this week? Seasonal foods, tips and recipes, updated weekly. (British, but mostly holds true for Ireland.)

Econatural.ie: an online Irish eco-store.

Ecoshop (www.ecoshop.ie) Irish eco-shop, now also online.

ENFO (www.enfo.ie) excellent source of environmental information. Established in 1990 by the Department of the Environment, Heritage and Local Government.

Edenbee (www.edenbee.com) Global swarming! The hive is a busy online community, buzzing with ideas to reduce our environmental footprint.

Ethical living (tinyurl.com/6ck8v8): sound advice on sustainable living, from the ethical living team at *The Guardian* newspaper.

Feasta (www.feasta.org) An old Irish lament asks, What will we do in the future without wood? The end of the forests has come . . . (*Cad a dhéanfaimid feasta gan adhmad? /Tá deireadh na gcoillte ar lár* . . .) This collective organisation works to save the trees, and build a sustainable future. Undertakes research, organises events and is open to membership.

Greenbox.ie Eco-tourism activities and accommodation across the six 'Greenbox' counties (Fermanagh, Leitrim, Cavan, Sligo, Donegal and Monaghan).

Green Me (greenme.ie) straight-talking green lifestyle tips and advice, news and views.

Green Pages (greenpages.ie) directory of Irish green products and services, plus articles on everything from ethical investments to fair-trade food. Run by Co-op Ireland Media Network Limited.

Green Wiki (green.wikia.com) aims to be the Wikipedia for environmental topics.

Green Drinks (url.ie/tdg) meets the first Tuesday of every month in the South William Bar (52 South William Street, Dublin 2), 6pm to 8pm. Coming soon to a town near you.

Green Business (www.greenbusiness.ie) National Waste Prevention Programme, a free service, offering advice, telephone helpline and even a visit to help Irish businesses go green and reduce waste.

Grist (www.grist.org) environmental news and commentary with a pinch of organic sea salt. US-based, but none the worse for that.

Guardian Environment Network (www.guardian.co.uk/environment/network) the best 'green' websites from around the world.

Happy Planet Index (www.happyplanetindex.org) How happy are you? Take the 'happy planet' questionnaire, and see how you compare.

Irish Environmental Network (www.ien.ie) broad network of 27 environmental NGOs.

Man in Seat 61 (seat61.com) for those who prefer to travel by train or boat.

New Scientist environment blog (www.newscientist.com/blog/environment) short, sharp and to the point, and includes Fred's Footprint (from veteran journalist Fred Pearce).

One Hundred Months (onehundredmonths.org) in August 2008, international agencies reckoned we had only 100 months before planet Earth reached the climate-change tipping point. At the time of going to press, it is 96 months and counting down. Join, and make every month count.

Organic Centre (www.theorganiccentre.ie): runs workshops on organic horticulture, green building, alternative energy and artisan food production from its base in County Leitrim.

Organic Guide to Ireland (www.organicguide.ie) the definitive guide to organic products and services for sale in Ireland. Book and website from the Organic Centre and the Soil Association.

Power of One (www.powerofone.ie) energy-saving tips and advice. From the Dept. of Communications, Marine and Natural Resources.

PriceWatch (www.irishtimes.com/pricewatch) Consumer affairs, cost comparisons, and an eye on the price of things, each Monday in *The Irish Times*.

Slow Food Ireland (www.slowfoodireland.com) news and events, on food as it should be.

Stop Climate Chaos (www.stopclimatechaos.ie) campaigning coalition of Irish NGOs.

Sustainability Institute (www.sustainability.ie): publishes *Sustainability* magazine, runs short courses and offers consultancy in construction and installation.

Sustainable Energy Ireland (www.sei.ie) grants for greener homes and renewable energy conversions, advice on energy efficiency, and support for new projects. Ireland's national energy agency.

Sustainable Ireland (www.sustainable.ie) a useful portal to Cultivate, The Village and related organisations.

Tap tips (www.taptips.ie) Don't waste water! Ways to save – at home, at work and in the garden. From your local authority.

Transition Culture (transitionculture.org) life after peak oil . . . Sustainability ideas from Rob Hopkins, who developed interesting projects in Kinsale and west Cork; now back in England.

Tree Hugger (www.treehugger.com) great web magazine packed with news, views, reviews and tips. US-based, but with a global reach.

The Village (www.thevillage.ie) Ireland's first eco-village, now being built in Cloughjordan, County Tipperary.

Water Footprint (www.waterfootprint.org) calculate your water footprint, or find out about the water footprint of various products and countries (no data yet for the Irish Republic). The University of Twente (Netherlands), with the UNESCO-IHE Institute for Water Education.

You Control Climate Change
(www.climatechange.eu.com) Turn down, switch off, walk. The European Commission's climate change campaign, with tips on what individuals can do to help bring it under control.

Your personal eco-footprint (www.ecofoot.org) calculate your eco-footprint. (You may have to pretend you live in the USA or Australia, but more countries are being added all the time.)